Blockchain

How to use the Hidden Economy to Your Advantage

The information herein is offered for informational purposes solely, and is universal as so. The presentation of the information is without contract or any type of guarantee assurance.

The trademarks that are used are without any consent, and the publication of the trademark is without permission or backing by the trademark owner. All trademarks and brands within this book are for clarifying purposes only and are the owned by the owners themselves, not affiliated with this document.

Table of Contents

Introduction

I want to thank you and congratulate you for purchasing *Blockchain: How to Use the Hidden Economy to Your Advantage*.

I have had a fascination with blockchain currencies for many years. When Bitcoin first rose to prominence, it fascinated me that so much value was being created out of nothing other than the faith that the currency will one day be worth something. This is the key the blockchain currencies – the value is determined by the faith that people have in the adoption of that currency. This is why Bitcoin currently has the largest capitalization; it is the most well known, widely accepted and easily made liquid.

I thought that I had arrived late to the world of cryptocurrencies, destined to be an observer and never a participant. Three years ago I decided that I would get involved in some lesser known currencies to see if I could turn a profit from mining for myself. To my surprise, I found that I could make decent income by merely setting up a few mining machines of my own. The key was in how I setup the machines, the parts used and the type of currency that I was mining. Also important was the timing of when I cashed out.

The goal of this book is to walk you through blockchain technology, what it's used for and how you can start making money quickly by obtaining some yourself. By the time you have completed this book you will have a fundamental understanding of blockchain currencies, know which currencies are good for mining, have a guide to get you started in building your mining farm, and know exactly what to look for to cash out at the optimal time for maximum profit.

You may have thought that the time has passed to get invested in blockchain technologies, but the truth is that there is still plenty of money to be made. Start reading and soon you will know how you can turn this exciting technology into profit for you and your family.

Victor Ashmore

Chapter 1: The Technology That Powers Cryptocurrencies

The Blockchain as Gold

Blockchain is a term that you might not be too familiar with, but chances are you've heard of the origin of the technology before. If you've ever stumbled across a news article about 'Bitcoin' then you are indeed at least familiar with blockchain. To truly understand the utility of blockchain as the underlying technology behind Bitcoin, you have to understand the intentions of the Bitcoin project.

The United States, and in fact the world economy, relies on the underpinning faith in the value of currency. This complex idea can be explained quite simply with a single U.S. dollar. A U.S. dollar has an assigned value to it, and we believe that this value is redeemable by nearly every vendor on Earth. It is this faith in the currency that gives the dollar its value. For many in the 21st century, they see this system as fundamentally flawed. The underlying value of the dollar is not a material good – it can be exchanged for everything but it is not pegged to a specific item. The value of a dollar is dependent on how many dollars are in circulation. This number, the total amount of currency on the market, is itself decided by the Federal Reserve Bank. Essentially, it is these very few people that decide the value of the dollars in our pockets. On a whim, and depending on the total supply of money, they can change the purchasing power of the dollars that we already have. For some, this idea is troublesome.

Prior to the 'on faith' system that came to true prominence in the 1970s, the United States and many other countries used the 'gold standard' system. This is a term that you might be familiar with, and in concept it is far easier to understand. The value of the dollar is merely a placeholder for the gold that it backs. We can print more money, but the gold that backs it is a finite resource. This disengages human medaling and in theory could lead to more stable and reasonable inflation.

The gold standard has many, many drawbacks, and there is hardly a mainstream economist alive that would vouch for it being a superior system to the one that we currently use, however the gold standard and the belief that it is a better system is the foundational idea behind blockchain technology.

What Exactly Is a Blockchain?

Blockchain technology allows Bitcoin to mimic a finite resource like gold, except it does so in the form of a digital currency. This combines the idea of value through a finite resource with all of the advantages of the digital age – rapid transmission, easier accesses to information, and the ability to truly decentralize the currency. One of the foundational concepts of Bitcoin is that there is no central bank. Access to information is spread evenly through all users of Bitcoin, and obtaining Bitcoin is given an equal chance to each and every participant to the currency. Blockchain technology facilitates each and every one of these goals.

Blockchain technology allows the decentralized distribution of Bitcoin, as well as keeping track of all transactions and the total number of coins in circulation. The 'chain' that it refers to is the data that accompanies each and every Bitcoin that is mined, as well as each and every transaction.

This idea can seem pretty complicated, but it can be explained quite easily. Imagine you and three of your friends all had a magic sheet of paper. Anything you wrote on this sheet of paper would be copied onto the other three sheets. You can't write something without it appearing on the copies that your friends have, as well as your friends can't write anything without it showing up on your sheet of paper. Now say that you used this sheet of paper to keep track of how much money you and your friends were lending to each other. Even if your other two friends aren't there when you lend one friend money, the other two will still know about it. With blockchain technology it is easy to see what was written on the sheet of paper and who wrote it. This means that you cannot cheat your friends and your friends cannot cheat you. They cannot perform an action without everyone becoming aware of it.

This is a large oversimplification, but you can see that we do not need a centralized bank to keep track of all transactions because included on each and every dollar is each and every other transaction that has ever happened in the past. This allows cooperation among many different people that don't know each other, and builds the foundation for trust that cannot be cheated or ruined through a single cheating actor.

What Purpose Does Blockchain Technology Serve?

As the technology underpinning Bitcoin and other cryptocurrencies, it allows all users to be aware of the actions of other users, including when, and this is arguably the most important aspect of blockchain technology, when another Bitcoin is 'mined.' No user can manipulate the currency by creating any out of thin air. Other users would see that they tried to manipulate the total amount in circulation and so executing such thievery is impossible.

Knowing that cryptocurrencies area a stand in for gold, we refer to the creation of Bitcoin and other currencies as 'mining' – just like mining gold. The action itself however, could not be any more different. Bitcoin and other cryptocurrencies mimic gold in many ways, starting with how many become available. If we think about gold, the amount of gold that is mined out of the Earth becomes less and less over time. We have found the large deposits of gold and if we were to graph the total amount of gold found year over year over a long time, we would see what looks like a downward heading parabola. We start with a steadily increasing slope till we hit the maximum, and then quickly follow a line downward as the gold gets harder to mine.

Cryptocurrency mimics the difficulty in finding gold by providing complex math equations. Think about solving these math equations as the equivalent of doing back breaking labor digging for gold. With digital currencies however, the agents finding the valuable material are computers. Users all have access to the same math equations, and they all try to solve them at the same time. Whoever solves the equation gets the coin. Because of the blockchain recording the same data for everyone, it means that for the computer that solves the equation and gets the coin, this is confirmed by every other computer also 'mining'. As time goes on, these math equations are programmed to get more and more difficult, mimicking the difficulty in mining for gold over time. There is only a finite amount of Bitcoins that will ever be produced, and nearly all cryptocurrencies operate under the same rule; they all wish to be a digital form of the gold standard in action.

How It *Really* Works

The previous sections help explain how blockchain technology works, but those early analogies will only take us so far. It's important to note the real world usage of blockchain technology like in Bitcoin. While the wallet that holds your cash only has one storage compartment for bills, your wallet for Bitcoin would have two very separate compartments. One is your private compartment, or 'private key' and the other is your public compartment, or 'public key'. Your private key is used to send money to other people, and it verifies that you are indeed the owner of the currency. The public key is used to view an address, the current balance and the owner's past transactions.

Let's say for example that you wish to send some Bitcoin to a friend, to send money you would prove ownership by providing a private key. The friend receiving money would take this key and verify the digital signature, in this case the key, and thus proves ownership of the corresponding private key. In other words, with the right address everyone can see transactions and balance data, but the right to move money from an account can only be done with the private key. Each transaction is then broadcasted to every computer in the Bitcoin network and is recorded in the blockchain. Again, the brilliance of this system cannot be understated – transactions are known to definitely have taken place because the public ledger is available to each and every computer on the Bitcoin network. They must all look at this data; the keys associated with the transaction, and agree that the transaction took place. This is the technical reason for why you do not need a centralized party to monitor transactions – each and every person on the network is that third party, in a practical sense, and ensuring the validity of the transaction.

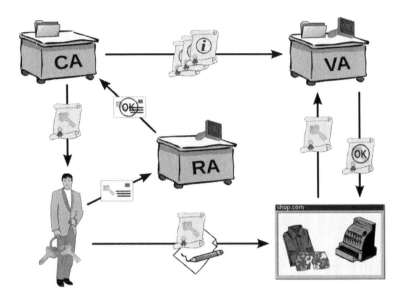

This above diagram shows the exact manner in which a private key can be used to purchase goods. The spender owns the cryptocurrency with the digital signature verification on the transaction. The spender has sufficient cryptocurrency in his or her account: checking every transaction against spender's account ('public key') in the ledger to make sure that he or she has a sufficient balance to complete the transaction.

The focus of the blockchain is to provide a system with no central control. This ensures the system cannot be shut down or changed by any single party. It enables the users of the network to know that they can safely use the network without the rules changing. Powering the decentralization is an ever-increasing capacity for verifying new blocks in the blockchain – the complicated math equations that facilitate the creation of new Bitcoins. As of this writing, there are nearly 1 quintillion (a billion billions) hashes per second going into Bitcoin proof-of-work to validate the blockchain.

Chapter 2: Why Are Cryptocurrencies Disrupting the Financial World?

Blockchain is gaining a lot of attention recently as innovative individuals are noticing that blockchain is not just a simple account ledger. Its applications are far wider than just digital currency, and instead its core characteristics of being secure, transparent and decentralized could revolutionize many industries. Blockchain can be implemented to change industry processes and cause major disruptions on existing business models because of how we conduct business transactions. There is an existing hierarchy of banks and credit processors that are threatened by blockchain currencies. They risk losing their main line of business as individuals flock to cryptocurrencies in the long run. This is not something that is likely to happen in the next two or three years, but in ten or twenty it is conceivable that the adaption rate of cryptocurrencies far exceeds the currency of any one nation.

You must know why blockchain currencies are valuable to understand when to sell them. In the next chapter you will see the primary mechanism in which you will be making money. Here, I would simply like to illustrate why your coinage will be gaining in value – what makes the currency so popular and why you might want to hold onto some currency.

Security
Where is your money the most secure? You might say the bank or in a mutual fund. You could argue for the stock market or government treasury bonds. It is doubtful that you would say your pocket or your mattress; after all, this is historically where the most disadvantaged have kept their

money. In 2016 and looking forward, it is no longer true that your money is most safely kept in a bank. The reasoning for this is simple; money that is stored online can be accessed online. By keeping your money online you open up the chance of more theft from your accounts. If you follow this logic, then all electronic accounts are more dangerous than keeping cash on your persons or in your home. This is one of the major driving factors for why cryptocurrencies are so popular. It offers a level of security greater than any other currency on the market, but can also be transferred digitally to any party in the world; it has features of all of the best aspects of currencies without any of the negatives.

Thinking about cryptocurrencies as cash is the best way to frame why they are so secure. The money that you have on you is far more secure than the money in a bank account. Granted the security at the bank is much greater, but only in the physical sense. By having your money stored in a digital location online, with no physical backup, a hacker can steal your money in a variety of ways. They can gain your identify and ring up false charges, or they can transfer money from your bank account to theirs. A scam that was recently publicized included a group that was pushing money to ATMs, allowing the scammers to simply steal cash from people's bank accounts.

In a pure digital sense, a bank has nearly an infinite number of entry points. Compare this to your home or your wallet, where you would physically need to be in the same location and have knowledge of where the money is kept before a thief can steal it. This is exactly how it functions with blockchain. Your physical funds are all stored digitally, online, and this information is shared across the world. What notifies others that the money is indeed yours is the encryption key that goes along with your wallet. The only way to a thief to steal your money is if they gain this encryption key – as long as this password is safe, it is impossible for someone to steal cryptocurrency from your persons. In this way, blockchain technologies serve to offer the immediacy and easy transfer of currency, the same as large banks with your digital accounts, with all of the safety of having your money on you at all times.

Speculation

Perhaps you have heard of FOREX markets. These are the currency exchanges of the world. Here speculators bet on currencies, buying and selling currency pairs dozens of times each and every day. It is just one factor in the complicated system that determines the exchange rate of currencies. These speculators are betting on whether or not a currency will increase or decrease in value. By the mere speculation on a currency, a currency's value could drop significantly.

Take for example the recent case with Mexico towards the end of 2016. When it was in limbo whether or not Donald Trump would win the American presidency, the Mexican Peso would fluctuate rapidly in price. This was all based on what the growing news story was at the time. If there was news about Donald Trump doing better in the polls then the currency would go down and if there was news that he was doing poorly the currency would go back up. A key component that is missed about this is that the currency fluctuation actually has nothing to do with what Donald Trump was saying about Mexico – it is instead had everything to do with how traders were reacting to Donald Trump's words. By simply signaling that Mexico might do worse in the future, speculators sold the Mexican Peso and the value overall dropped very quickly.

Blockchain currencies aren't entirely immune to speculation. In fact, right now it is a major hurdle for digital currencies. The main problem is in the exchange of a blockchain currency for a currency issued by a government. Right now this is a necessary step for many currency traders. You simply cannot buy the same number of goods that you can with a digital currency as you can a physical currency backed by a government. For tips to the grocery store, you will need to convert money to cash. The true problem is that the market changes from highly liquid to solid in a matter of a few hours or days. The number of places that you can exchange online coinage for real currencies is limited, and so they need to cover their bottom line from rapid currency fluctuations. In the end, the customer ends up getting the short end of the stick, ending up with far less in real currency than they should be getting for their digital currency.

Blockchain based currencies will become more stable with time. You can see that right now the problem exists when converting from cryptocurrencies to regular government backed money. In this exchange the rates vary wildly. The main way in which this problem will be solved is when cryptocurrencies become more widely used in stores. The true value of cryptocurrency is almost exclusively in speculation. This means that most that have digital currency opt to hold onto it for the long term. This is wise, as the value of cryptocurrencies tomorrow is going to be worth far more than what they are worth today. For you, you will want to hold onto your digital currencies for as long as possible, only selling if you absolutely need to, or if you want some immediate profit up front.

Government Intervention

Traditional currencies fall under the supervision of government bureaucracies. These antiquated agencies regulate currencies by determining the total amount that is available in circulation, as well as determining the overall interest rates of the currency from common lenders. This gives the government a decent amount of control in their own currency. As you read from chapter one, this is a significant change from how governments operated when they were backed by the gold standard. With all of the good that comes from being able to control a currency within a country's borders, there also come many major problems as well.

After the 2008 financial crisis, the interest in cryptocurrencies rose significantly. Some of this had to do with the technology coming into its own at the time, but a lot of that had to do with how people were viewing the government's actions on how they were handling the U.S. dollar. For years after the financial crisis, the government rose inflation on the dollar significantly, through a procedure called 'quantitative easing'. This is fancy term for pumping cash into the economy, but with a plan to eventually siphon that same money out. This is supposed to reduce the overall effect of inflation, and to some degree it did work, however the cryptocurrencies that you will deal with will not have any of these issues. They will be immune from government intervention.

Being completely immune from government control, cryptocurrencies will not suffer from inflation. You learned in chapter one that the design of cryptocurrencies is based off of gold – the original tender that is immune from human controlled inflation. What this will means for you as a trader is that the value of your currency can only ever go up. It rewards those that hold onto their money instead of spending it on goods and services. This in turn only raises the value of cryptocurrencies. Think about it this way; if the money in your pocket was depreciating, you would be incentivized to spend it as soon as possible. This is true for you and everyone else that is using the same currency. For cryptocurrency, the exact opposite situation arises. It is more profitable for you and for everyone else to hold onto the money in their pockets, increasing the value of the currency over time. This is just another reason why it is always worth holding onto your currency; the less sense it makes to use the currency outside of speculation just increases how quickly the value of the currency rises.

A One-To-One Transaction

It is my belief that the most significant advantage of cryptocurrencies comes in how transactions are handled when using digital money. In essence, the big change is that there is no third party credit processor. All transactions can take place between just two parties. This may sound like a minor advantage, but the applications for what a cryptocurrency can do are simply endless when you think about the switch between credit swaps and cash swaps.

Digital currencies function as electronic cash. This means that transactions that you make online are completely anonymous. In the large hash file for a currency, you will have the record that you gave someone money, but there is no memo and the only way that someone can tell who you are is if they match up your wallet identification with who provided the payment. These anonymous transactions that involve no third party payment processor are monumentally important as we move forward into the twenty first century. The rise of the sharing economy has seen a huge boom for companies that act as middlemen between those doing the labor and those seeking services. With cryptocurrencies, this dynamic is set to change – there will be no need for a third party processor. The exchange can happen simply between two parties, increasing the value of the work done. If the adoption rate continues at current trends, what this will mean is quite stupendous – the value of cryptocurrencies will rise as the desire for them grows. People will want digital currencies because they can get cheaper services. This might sound a little complicated, but think about it this way: have you ever paid cash to someone for a cheaper product than if you were paying on credit? It is the same premise, and is the same reason why $10 of cash is more valuable than $10 of credit. As more people start to see the value of cryptocurrencies, and as they try and get their hand on this money, the value will rise and miners like you will be doing better.

Summary

In this chapter we've covered the fundamental reason why digital currencies will continue to rise in value, and why they will continue to find more and more uses over time. I want you to note something; do not sell your digital currencies or use them in exchange for goods or services. Currencies will always have more value over time, much like gold. Using them in the moment is always going to be a bad idea if you are thinking about cryptocurrencies as an investment. It will be more and more tempting to use digital currencies as more vendors start accepting it as a form of payment, but the problem is this is the very type of action that makes the money in your pocket more valuable. As you start to see digital currencies used more and more, think about it as a way of knowing that the money you have is appreciating, instead of a sign that you should use the money on goods now.

Chapter 3: Making Blockchain Work for You

Where You Will Make a Profit

You should have a good understanding of how blockchain currencies work and why they are due to appreciate in value. You have a good knowledge base of both the technical and the economic theory behind these digital currencies. Now it is time to move on to how you will make money from digital currencies. Chapters four and five will discuss the practical knowledge you need for help setting up your mining operation, but for now let's cover the basic strategy for how you will be earning a profit.

Your strategy for making profit is one of the oldest in history, speculation. This might sound like a dirty word, but in essence you are an early investor who is getting involved by merely buying or gaining the currency to sell it at a later time. You are going to be among those that make the value of cryptocurrencies rise. In the last chapter you learned about how speculators are a fundamental problem for traditional forms of currency, so it's important to address why this is not actually a problem for digital currencies. With digital currencies you will be speculating on the currency itself, not on its value in relation to other money. The main difference here is that in FOREX trading a currency is always traded in relation to a different currency. I gave an example of how the Mexican Peso fluctuated in value many times during 2016. This was not an isolated change in the value of the currency; it was in conjunction with how the U.S. dollar was changing. The dollar was rising in value compared to Peso, forcing the Peso to drop.

The type of speculation that you are working with on digital currencies is being an early adopter of cryptocurrency. That is technically the value that you are adding to gain profit at the end of your venture. That is essentially all of the 'work' that you are doing. How you actually gain the cryptocurrencies is a matter of your investment and that is where you will break a sweat, and have to potentially open your wallet. The deciding factor in why you are going to make a greater profit in comparison to your fellow man is a factor of how well you understand where cryptocurrencies fit into the world. By knowing when to sell your currency, you will be position yourself to make the most profit. This is what is going to decide the great investors from others – this is where you will need to have an edge to make the most profit.

What You Need to Lookout For

The validating part of the blockchain is extremely resource heavy and there is a real problem of how many blocks the blockchain can produce to carry on recording. This problem has not been solved yet and is one that has several different solutions available. There has been a recent push for a different standardization of how this information is hashed. The problem is that with all things related to cryptocurrencies, it would need to have a consensus by the entire community. Right now, especially with the more popular currencies, there are too many big players that have an advantage in the way that it is currently setup. I think that it is doubtful that the hashing system will change anytime in the future, but it is something that you will want to be on the lookout for. The primary concern is that someone will use a change in the hashing system to take advantage of how the money is mined. They will then use this for their own purposes and make money while the rest of the traders ultimately lose.

The only way to avoid this issue is to follow the news on the cryptocurrencies that you trade. Remember that if you get involved in this type of investment that it is an active one, and something that you cannot just invest in and walk away. You will need to consistently follow the events of your currency and be ready to back out at the time that is most profitable for you. The likely driving factors of this do not come from the currencies themselves, but rather outside intervention. It is in the hashing system where the one weakness imbued to cryptocurrencies exists. As long as you are diligent in your awareness of how the hashing system works, or rather if it has been changed, you should always end on the more profitable side of investors.

The Cryptocurrencies You Should Mine

You've heard of a few cryptocurrencies, but you probably aren't aware that there are a decent number of options available today that look promising. Below is a list of the most in demand currencies today (based on market capitalization). Anything with a * is one that I would recommend mining. The * currencies have great potential and you will be a relatively early adopter for mining. The exception to this is Bitcoin, which is well adopted but difficult to mine. I suggest having one computer mine Bitcoin purely because it has the highest present day value.

1. Bitcoin*
2. Ripple
3. Litecoin*
4. Bitshares
5. Darkcoin
6. Nxt*
7. Dodgecoin

8. MaidSafeCoin*
9. Stellar
10. Paycoin

Chapter 4: Beginner's Guide to Mining

Mining Principles

There are only two ways that you can get any cryptocurrency; you can either buy it or you can mine it. While it is conceivable that you could buy some number of cryptocurrencies and hold onto them until they appreciate, it is far more likely that you are interested in mining them yourself. This has grown to be quite a competitive field, but once the initial hardware investment is made, it can certainly pay off quite well in the long run. What you will need to get started is a computer and the shareware software for calculating hashes in a given currency. In this chapter I will walk you through everything that you need to know about mining to get started. I am estimating that you have some level of computer literacy, but for the most part things will be simple enough that even a novice will know where to get started.

You could use your current laptop or desktop, but chances are your computer is not fast enough to get a good number of hashes. You might realize half a Bitcoin over the course of five years on a traditional Intel laptop for example. For years the equipment that you needed was quite expensive, but as advances in computing continue to take hold, the total cost has dropped significantly. Realistically, you will need to have three or four computer systems running 24/7 to truly see a profit in any sort of good time frame.

Your initial investment on each computer is not that large; approximately five to six hundred dollars per machine should do it. This will cover a basic computer with a weak CPU and fairly powerful GPU (more on this in a moment). Remember that you will not need a monitor for your computer systems as the process is entirely automated. You will plug a computer into a monitor to run the setup process but once everything is set, you can unplug the monitor and hook it into another computer system.

Mining on desktop computers is the basic principle for how you will be making money, but really quick I want to illustrate the type of horsepower that you will need to make this work. If you have ever had a virus on your computer that has slowed down the entire system to a very large degree, it is likely that you were involved in a Bitcoin mining operation. A hacker installed software on your computer remotely and is using the power from your machine to create hashes for themselves. This is actually a fairly common way that some hackers get into mining Bitcoins – they distribute the processing power required across a wide network of computers that are infected with malware. I make this point to show that the machines that you will be mining on will only be used for mining. The processing power required makes doing most other tasks on the machines at the same time not realistic.

Necessary Equipment

There are six essential building blocks that you will need to source to create a small 'farm' for mining. You will need a CPU, GPU, Memory, Storage, Power Supply and Motherboard. You may also want a case to house all of these components, but it is not actually necessary. This is doubly true if you are building several machines that will be next to each other. The rest of this chapter is dedicated to going over how each component will play its role in helping you mine, and what you should spend money on and what is not worth your time.

You might have some concerns about not being able to build your own computer for mining. I want you to rest assured that building your own computer is quite easy. For mining, you are building a full computer system, or rather one that has all of the main components. There are dozens of tutorials for how to do this online. What you want to be on the lookout for is instruction materials basing on 'gaming' computers. In essence, your machine is going to house many similar parts to a computer designed to run videogames; you will just have some greater concern about certain parts and worry less about others. Tutorials based on building a gaming PC covers all of the basics of how to assemble a machine. It really is quite like building with Lego – that is, anyone can do it. You simply must learn and the resources are quite plentiful to help you.

CPU and GPU

You might be extremely knowledgeable about computers but still be confused about the terms 'CPU' and 'GPU'. There is little doubt that you've at least heard of one of these, but to underhand exactly what they do and how they fit into mining is important. These are going to be your primary profit drivers. Making sure that you have the suitable hardware and that you are investing in the right parts will mean more profit for you in the long run. The CPU stands for the central processing unit, and the GPU stand for the graphics processing unit. Perhaps unintuitive, but the GPU will be a far more important component than the CPU for your mining operation.

The CPU is the main processing unit for your computer. It handles all of the basic calculations that run your operating system. You already know that this is not the major component that will work on mining for you, but it doesn't mean that you can cheap out on this component either. The CPU is responsible for handing off instructions to your GPU, and without a fast enough cycle it will start to be the limiting factor for how fast your GPU can hash. You will want to shoot for at least a modern I-5 processor from Intel. You could opt for an AMD processor, which tend to be cheaper, but I wouldn't recommend it. It is not because the speed is so vastly different for mining, but rather that you can get away with an older generation Intel processor and you simply can't do the same with AMD. You will need the latest processors from AMD to be able to mine effectively. For either processor that you choose, you won't need to worry about the clock speed. If you don't know what this is, then don't worry – if you do know what this is, then simply do not adjust it. For the cooling of your CPU, you can get away with a $20-$30 aftermarket air cooler. I don't advise investing in a liquid cooling solution for the CPU – it simply isn't worth the effort or maintenance when it comes to mining. You will be more than capable with just the air cooled solution. You should expect that each main processor you buy is going to be between $180-$250. You can get a processor for more or for less but this is the price range that will get the job done for mining. Remember that the most important part of the processor is not speed, but just stability and heat concerns. This the basis for my recommendation of going with Intel processors; they tend to be more reliable.

The GPU is going to be the far more important component for your mining machines. The GPU is the processor that handles all of the graphics that seen on your display. You should note that most laptops do not have dedicated GPUs and that is why there are so poor at mining cryptocurrencies. For graphics, laptops simply offload the calculations to the CPU, which are capable of rending videos and the operating system, but little more. Even if your laptop

28

does have a discrete video card, there is little doubt that it wouldn't be very powerful.

This will be a major part of your mining computer so you won't want to skimp on price. You can expect this component to run you around $200 per GPU. In the next chapter dedicated to strategies you will learn about the different models and pick the one that best serves your needs, but for now know that what you care about is the number of cores and the clock speed on the GPU. These are the most basic factors that will determine the overall hashing ability of your machine, and is the reason why GPUs are much more important than CPUs in this regard. GPUs come loaded with many more cores that handle small calculations. This is a byproduct of being a part designed to render video graphics, like in games. Because miners are interested in buying GPUs specifically for mining, the costs have become abnormal in regard to what models are in demand. Some of the leading video cards in sales are not very good at rendering videogames at all but instead are top sellers because they are good at mining.

There are several factors in play for deciding what GPU is right for you. Aside from the number of cores and clock speed, there is the architecture and power to be concerned about. These are all factors that you will learn more about in the next chapter; these are the primary drivers in what makes a good GPU for mining. What is the best selling model of GPU for mining Bitcoin might not be an ideal fit for your purposes. This is a multifaceted problem, including cost, power, and wattage requirements. As a final note on GPUs for this section, it is often times going to be beneficial to buy a used unit instead of a brand new one. GPUs are binary devices in that they either work or they don't, there is very little room for a failing GPU that only works part of the time (this is usually a heat problem and not an issue with the board itself). This binary state of GPUs opens up the number of places where you can buy a board. It is not like buying a used car, in that for the most part you don't care about the overall condition; you just need to know if it works right now.

Memory

The memory, RAM (random access memory) of your mining computer is important, but it is not a crucial factor that will make your break your rig. In general you will want to have around 8GB of ram. You can certainly get away with 4GB or 6GB, but the costs are relatively low so an upgrade shouldn't be your largest problem. The only concern that you need to have is if the RAM is compatible with your motherboard. RAM is broken down into categories of DDR; the most current type of RAM is DDR4, however there is still a lot of DDR3 on the market. If you were to build a computer today, you would end up with one of these two types of RAM requirements. Simply make sure that you have at least 4GB and the RAM is compatible and you will be ready to go.

Storage

This is a component that I often see left out of other materials for creating mining machines. The storage is the component that houses all of the written information on your machine. This means that it is storing the hashing information and data about the cryptocurrency that is making its way to your wallet. The coins that are in your wallet will appear online, but you don't want to lose all of the native hashing data, just in case. This is a big in case because all miners will have a backup, but it would be handy to have the original hashing document. Aside from being where your data is stored, there is another reason why you will want to have a decent storage unit for your machine. The storage component is likely going to be the first part of your machine that breaks down. Your machine will need this part to run and will shut down immediately if it breaks.

You mainly have two options for how you want to store your data. These are the hard drive (HDD) and the solid state drive (SSD). You may have heard of both of these terms before. They are similar pieces of hardware but they function on a mechanical level very differently. There is also something called a 'hybrid' drive which has elements of an SSD and HDD. As a rule of thumb, go with HDDs but buy several. What I do in my own systems is I have two hard drives for each one of my mining machines. These hard drives are setup in a 'Raid' configuration. You will need to refer to the owner's manual for your motherboard to set this up properly, but what this does is have two hard drives connected with one constantly creating a backup of the other. This allows for one component to fail and for the other to take over immediately. It ensures that there is no downtime and that you do not lose any of your data.

I do not recommend that you buy SSDs or hybrid drives. They are simply not necessary for the purpose of mining cryptocurrencies. I have seen the argument before that their increased reliability makes them worthwhile, but I don't think the math quite works out. I've also seen that the power draw on these devices in less, adding to savings in electricity over time. You can't argue with this, but the draw is extremely small to begin with for storage devices. In the end, just use a hard drive and don't worry about the more expensive storage solutions.

Power Supply

The fixed cost of running a mining operation is the electricity bill that you will have to pay each month. The power supplies that you choose for your machines will be a determining factor in how large you can expect your bill to be. Perhaps more importantly however, a poor power supply can break an entire system, ruining all other components and ensuring that the machine never runs again. You will want to be careful in what power supply you choose to run in each of your machines. There are a couple guidelines that you can use; the power supplies should be gold rated and support at least 400 watts.

Power supplies are rated from bronze to platinum. There are all the rare power supplies that do not have a rating at all. This rating is extremely important for estimating the life expectancy of the part. A cheap power supply is the first component to break on a mining computer because the machine is running all the time. What the ratings mean is that the machine can output a certain percentage of the said wattage on the box. This is a little complicated and specific to computer parts, but the premise is that a 400 watt power supply never outputs 400 watts. It outputs closer to around 70% of 400 watts. Over time this percentage is going to drop, until eventually the power supply cannot output the necessary amount of power the computer needs. The rating is supposed to only determine the percentage that you can expect to get out of the power supply, but it also says quite a bit about the quality of a power supply. One that is not rated at all can easily fail within a year. One that is platinum rated can last five years without any problems.

You should expect to spend at least $50 per power supply unit. These devices can range heavily in price and it might be tempting to buy one that is not rated – you can find one of these for as cheap as $12-15 for example. You will want to avoid this for one reason; all power supplies fail, but how they fail is dependent on the build quality of the device. A poorly built power supply won't just break, it will light on fire. Bar that, it will knock out every component that it is hooked up to by providing too much power to all of the components. This means that you can knock out your memory, storage, CPU and GPU; all from buying a cheap power supply. It is better to be safe than sorry – spend a little more money and change out the power supply once every three years. This is about the longest that you want to have a power supply running, regardless of rating. Remember that you are using these machines in a nontraditional way; you are running at max power at all times. Normal computers were not designed to be running at full load all the time.

I have seen several people advocate using one large power supply to run multiple machines. I highly advise against doing this. It may cut some costs upfront, but it brings many issues. Even if it is a highly rated power supply, you are opening yourself up to more risk because of the high wattage requirements. You are also requiring some modifications to allow for the power supply to function with two main processor units – something that can be done but is never advised. Most importantly, if a power supply fails it can take every connected component out with it. This would be bad enough if it takes out one of your mining machines, but two would just be devastating.

Motherboard

The motherboard may not be the first component that you buy for your machine, but it should be the first part you plan around because it will dictate nearly every other component that can be used. If you are building a computer around a certain processor, you will need to make sure that the motherboard is a match. This component is important because it will dictate several other parts that you are going to use. For example, the brand of CPU that you buy for your machine will be entirely based on what motherboard you are using. A motherboard is either designed to be used with one company or the other, and can never be used with both. Along with this comes the model of processor that can be used. Your motherboard will have a 'socket' type that determines what type of processor will fit into this slot. This means that not all Intel processors work on motherboards approved for Intel – the motherboard only works with one particular socket type and not the others. The motherboard holds your computer together and will also provide the networking capability for your machine.

The motherboard will also determine the type of memory that you will use. As I stated before, the difference between DDR3 and DDR4 is not very substantial, and either will do just fine. Your motherboard will have explicit instructions for what type of RAM that it accepts. As long as you follow the included instruction manual, you will be fine.

There is one last consideration to take into account with your motherboard, and that is size. The more spaced out a motherboard is the less of an issue heat becomes. It is also easier to assemble a machine with a larger board. Overall, I suggest that you buy your motherboard based on price, but if this is your first time assembling a computer you might want to spring for a large size motherboard just to ensure that you have enough room to assemble your machine comfortably. You can expect this part to cost between $30 and $80. The price range is considerable here because of how frequently models are iterated on. Many of the features of these boards you do not care about, aside from the ones that are listed above. Always shoot for what is cheaper and you will do fine.

Operating System

You're probably familiar with Apple's operating system, OSX, and Microsoft's operating system, Windows. Both of these are suitable for mining cryptocurrencies; however the type of currency that you can mine will be determined by what operating system you have. Bitcoin for example can be mined on any operating system. Some lesser known currencies can only be mined on Windows. As a general rule, the most compatible operating system is Windows. A license for the most recent version of windows will run you around $100, making it a sizeable part of your investment in any one machine. You will want to avoid this and use Linux instead. Linux is an open source operating system based on the same kernel that powers Apple's operating system. There are enough cryptocurrencies that have miners for Linux that this will be your best value proposition.

To install Linux on one of your machines you will first need to get a copy. This is done easily enough by searching online for a version of Linux and following the instructions. All you will need is a USB storage device with around 4GB of space. This storage device won't be used for storing anything other than the Linux operating system, and can be used multiple times to install the OS on as many different machines as you would like.

One additional note on operating systems; do not use any operating system that is not 100% legitimate. There was a time when versions of Windows circulated online and could be activated without issue. This is no longer the case, and typically these 'free' versions of paid operating systems are a neat ploy to ruin a computer with malware. It's typically a version of Windows that doesn't receive any updates at the very least. It should be avoided at all costs. Simply either use Linux or pay for the Window's license.

What You Don't Need

You now know all of the components that you will need to buy and how they fit into mining. You may be thinking to yourself that you know computers have a lot of other components, and you would be right, but the problem is that no other components are going to be necessary for mining. They are in fact are all superfluous to what your goal is for each of the machines that you are going to build. This includes parts like CD/DVD readers, keyboards, mice and monitors. You will need a keyboard and mouse to interact with the computer during the setup phase, but once that is done you can disconnect the parts and still have the computer run. The same is true for the monitor. The moment you are done configuring the machine and have setup the mining software, you should disconnect the monitor. You can then use it on a different machine, or at the very least turn it off. Your main enemy in producing profit is the electricity that you use to create currency – every little bit helps, including turning off all your monitors.

Chapter 5: Strategies for Mining

The Fixed Cost

The electric company is your main enemy when it comes to creating profit through mining for cryptocurrency. The amount that you need to pay for generating any amount of currency is based on how much power went into the computation for that computer part. Accordingly, this chapter is dedicated to strategies to help you minimize the total amount of electricity that you need to mine. In the last chapter you learned about the basic components and got some tips and guidelines for what to buy. Here, I will be getting a little bit more specific, talking about what brands you should use and which ones to avoid.

The key to making a great profit through mining is to cut down on your costs, and the best way to do this is to be creative. You learned that hackers often plant malware on other computers for the purpose of having infected machines mine for cryptocurrencies. Although highly inefficient, for the hackers this is a great way to earn free money because they do not have to pay any of the associated power costs of the mining. While I don't suggest you do anything along the lines of these hackers, you will want to be creative in how you can save electricity.

AMD and NVidia

There are only two GPU makers that are competitive in the market today, NVidia and AMD. Buying GPUs for mining is one of the most difficult aspects of setting up your farm. You will need to compare three metrics – price, performance, and power draw. My suggestion for beginners is to use the RX470 by AMD. This card is less than $200 and is more than capable of getting the job done. The RX 400s series is the current line that AMD produces. Regardless of the card that you buy, you will want to use a 400 series model. The 480 is also an option, however the 470 is more in the sweet spot in terms of price and what you are using it for.

NVidia cards tend to be more expensive than AMD and they are not as great at mining blockchain currencies. That being said, they are also far more reliable, often operate at lower temperatures, and currently have the lowest power draw on the market. The main GPU that you will want to buy if you decide to go this route is the 1060; a great card that has an incredibly small power draw. All 900 series models are also decent to use for mining, but note that they use much more power than the 1000 line. Avoid the 700 series as this technology is too old and consumes too much power; there is no 800 series.

Thermal Paste

Assembling a desktop for mining is fairly straight forward and you should know which parts you need. Often what is under appreciated is the importance that thermal paste plays in reducing the costs of electricity over time. The hotter your CPU/GPU, the more expensive they are to run, and the faster they burn out. Thermal paste is the conduit between a processor and a cooling unit. All of the air that flows through a cooling unit interacts with the thermal paste, dissipating the heat from the processor. The more effective the thermal paste, the less heat. If you find that your systems are running hotter than they should, a likely factor is that you applied *too much* thermal paste to a processor. All you need is a light application to create a very thin layer. Usually a simple dot in the middle, and then spread it out when mounting the cooling unit on top. In terms of the paste itself, when you buy a processor it comes with a small amount of stock paste. You will not want to use this and instead opt for something like: Arctic Silver brand thermal paste. It's a bit more expensive but the reduction in the cost of power is enough to justify the purchase.

Monitoring the System

Your mining machines shouldn't have any monitors hooked up all the time. That being said, you will want to periodically monitor the temperature of each computer. There are a few components that you want to pay attention to. The reason why the temperature matters so much is that an increase in temperature will mean a greater power draw from your machine, typically from the cooling solution working harder, but more importantly you are going to burn out the parts faster. The cooler you can have your main components run, the longer each individual part is going to last.

The two main components that you will want to monitor are the GPU and CPU. You don't need to worry about the temperature of the RAM or motherboard, though many pieces of software will include these temperatures. As a general rule of thumb, you want to keep your CPU temperatures below 75 degrees Celsius and your GPU temperatures below 85 degrees Celsius. Running at or below these temperatures, you can expect hardware to last for around four years when in use 24/7. There is a lot of disagreement around these temperatures, and you will see some proponents of running at temperatures far below these. I have found that the temperatures of 75 and 85 degrees Celsius are the perfect combination of easily attainable, and provide enough life in the parts to make money back on investment.

To monitor the temperature for your CPU and GPU, you should download 'CoreTemp' for your CPU and 'MSI Afterburner' for your GPU. There are many other monitoring solutions available, but these are the ones that I personally use. You should note that sometimes monitoring software will not display the same temperature as another piece of software. This has to do with where the software is getting the reading from. What you care about is the actually 'core' temperature of the hardware, not the ambient temperature around the hardware. I suggest that you have this software running 24/7 while you mine, and then check the maximum temperature for both components about once every three or four days. Over the course of a few weeks you will notice that this temperature goes up a little bit, but as long as it stays below the values above then you are in the clear.

Dust Is an Enemy

You will notice the temperature on your components creep up over time because of dust. Computers, particularly desktops, are great attractors of dust. It is impossible to keep one running without getting a significant amount of dust buildup over time. You will want to clean out your machines once a month, *at a minimum*. This increases if you have pets, where you should clean components once a week. To do a quick cleanup of the dust in the machine, use compressed air to blow dust from around the openings of any fans or cooling units. You will never be able to get every bit of dust out of each machine, but you should be able to get pretty close. Since you are doing this regularly, I suggest that you buy a compressed air unit for PCs. Unlike a compressed air can, this is a device that plugs into an outlet and has both suction and blowing capabilities to get rid of dust. It may seem like a large investment up front, but compressed air cans are not cheap, and over the course of the first year this will cost you less money.

In addition to cleaning components once a month with air, you will also want to do a thorough cleaning job once every six to eight months. For this, you will be dismantling each one of your major units and reapplying thermal paste on the necessary components. Typically this means applying thermal paste to the CPU, but if you also have an aftermarket cooler for your GPU, you will need to reapply it on that as well. When doing a full clean, make sure that you also clean out the power supply unit. This is very important as it is a closed unit. It can be hard to see inside and you cannot dismantle it yourself. Your best bet is to take a vacuum to the side of the power supply unit to suck out all of the dust. This is a *huge factor* in the power draw of your unit. A power supply that is full of dust is going to be less efficient than a clean unit.

Static

Static is not going to increase the total amount of heat from your mining farm, but it will play a factor in maintenance and assembly. Static is one of the hazards of working with computers, and is the reason why computers typically come encased. While you don't need a case for each of your mining machines, you will want to make sure that every time you touch a unit you are 'grounded'. That is, you should touch a piece of metal that is separate from the computer unit. If you touch a computer component and send a bit of static electricity through it, it could be enough to short the unit. This is fairly rare, but can certainly happen if you are not careful.

You can avoid this altogether by wearing an anti-static band when working on your machines, but I have found that this isn't really necessary. All you need to lookout for is making sure that you have grounded yourself before you do

41

any maintenance, and that you are not doing anything to make yourself more prone to static. For example, try not to walk on carpet before touching your mining machines. Most importantly, don't wear socks when working on a computer, and try and keep away clothing and hair that dangle into computer components.

Consider Heat and Different Cooling Solutions

Heat will be a major concern of yours as you start to get involved in mining. Even if you are only running two or three systems, the heat generated from mining adds up over time. For most, this is only a minor concern, but I wanted to point it out here in case you live in a warm climate. For example, I have a partner that works outside of Houston – the additional equipment that they need to ensure that the computer systems that mine do not fry is immense. The colder the climate, the more you can cut back on expensive cooling equipment for your mining PCs. There are three ways in which you will avoid heat from being a problem.

The first way to diminish the effects of heat is to get hardware that is power efficient. This means far more than just consuming less electricity, it also means producing far less heat. The more heat that your systems produce, the greater the chance that they will start to 'throttle' themselves; that is purposefully slow down to avoid damage. For what you are trying to accomplish, you want to make sure that clock speeds are running at maximum whenever possible.

The second way to avoid issues relating to heat is to operate machines in a cool environment. This is the most basic way of solving a heat problem, but note that how much of an effect this actually has is quite minimal. The ambient temperature of a room only has so much say on how much heat a computer system in going to produce. It ends up being far more of a problem when a room is hot – it does not solve the problem when the room gets cold. I mention this because it means that blasting the air conditioning is not a valid way of reducing the heat from a computer system. It is an extremely inefficient way of cooling a series of machines, and simply won't be as effective as the first and third methods for reducing heat. You should only assume that the environmental conditions are a net positive for your machines if they are operating in a room that is close to freezing. This is the only way in which environmental conditions even start to come close to conditions that will have a positive impact on heat. This is also where I will note that in a cold environment, the heat that is generated by your computer systems is a decent way to heat up a small to medium sized room. You may need to run your traditional heating system for less time if your mining setup is near where you stay in your home.

The third and most efficient way of reducing heating problem from mining system is through aftermarket cooling solutions. These are special 'coolers' that are slated on top of GPUs or CPUs to reduce the overall heat. They come in two variants, either liquid cooled or air cooled. Both have advantages and disadvantages, but overall liquid cooling wins out. While most of your computer system is something that you can setup yourself, you will want some help when installing these aftermarket coolers. This requires getting dangerously close to the main boards where the electronic components are kept. Handling these the wrong way could short circuit the boards and ruin the entire unit.

The fundamental difference between air cooled and liquid cooling solutions are the conductive material that runs through the processing unit of a computer. The way in which these devices are cooled is important – it illustrates the best type of setup that you can have for yourself. The GPU and CPU units cool by having the heat on the boards release into the air. All the liquid and air cooling solutions do is increase the amount of air that gets in contact with the heat from the circuits. This is true with the liquid cooling even though it might not seem that way – the liquid acts as a conduit for cool air to cool off the board of the processor. In terms of cost and ease of use, air coolers are far cheaper than liquid coolers. They are effective at cooling boards to a certain degree, and also produce less noise than liquid coolers. The most substantial difference is in the maintenance required. Liquid coolers have more points of failure and required maintenance. You will need to replace parts more often and doing so is frequently far more intensive work than doing something similar with an air cooler.

Be Creative with Where You Source Parts

Your go-to shops for computer parts will be major retailers like Best Buy, Newegg, Amazon, etc. The type of parts that you buy will die over time, but until the day they die they function just as well as the day they were created. What this means is, don't be afraid to buy used. Get creative with where you are buying your parts from. I have purchased several GPUs through Craigslist for great prices. The one thing you will want to be on the lookout for is if the part has been used to mine blockchain currencies. This puts serious wear and tear on the card, and while it won't' perform any differently while it works, it will likely fail much sooner too.

Chapter 6: Calculating Profitability

Bills Today and Predictions of Tomorrow

Calculating your profitability from mining cryptocurrency is difficult or rather, next to impossible. Anyone that tells you something different is lying. There are too many unknowns to truly figure out what your degree of profitability is going to be. The best way to try and figure out your profit margin is to cut down as much as possible on the costs of maintenance and electricity for your mining machines. You will also want to cash out at the right time and make sure that you are staying current what the types of currencies that you mine. As a basic rule, you want to be invested in at least two different currencies – this is to hedge your bets on which currencies will be more valuable in the future.

It is impossible to calculate the wattage/dollar amount in mining because profits are not realized until the currency is traded for a major currency backed by a government. You can't follow past trends on a currency either, as right now it is nothing but speculation with incredible price swings being a common occurrence. You will need to wait until there is some stability in the market to truly be able to calculate your total profit. There is a real chance that this stability is many years off, and almost certainly several currencies will fall before any major cryptocurrencies becomes mainstream. In the next chapter you will read about signs of when you should cash out, but right now know that it is impossible to calculate true profits and that the estimation that cryptocurrencies will be worth something one day is based on the usefulness of the technology and not any sort true value in the currency – the coins/dollars are worth nothing by themselves. If all of this sounds dim about potential profits in the present, don't worry.

I highly advocate cashing in your digital currencies when you are ready to seek a return on investment. Just be sure to hold onto some of each currency in case the value rises significantly in the future.

You will want to get involved in at least two currencies, as to hedge your bet for what will be successful. This does not mean that you won't have to be on the lookout for signs when to sell, but it means that you are diversifying your investment. If I were starting today, I would invest in one major currency and one budding currency. A good combo would be go to for Bitcoin and Nxt. Bitcoin is established and if it ever does fail, it will have several months of depreciation before being worth nothing. For Nxt, the current market cap is just shy of $15 million, but the foundational technology is the same as Bitcoin. There is evidence to suggest that it will be successful based on how difficult it will be for individuals to comprise the hashing system because of the existing framework. Investing in these two currencies is a good amount of diversification, and if you can't find profit in one, you almost certainly will be able to find profit in the other.

In the present, your primary concern is going to be on reducing power draw. Use all of the tips from chapter five to ensure that you are running your mining farm as efficiently as possible. Pay close attention to your electric bill and note when it gets more expensive – when it does, try and figure out why. Note that most electric companies do not have fixed rates on their wattage, meaning it is cheaper to run electronics at night than it is during the day. It is cheaper to operate your mining machines in the Fall and Spring than it is in the Summer and Winter. It will be worth it to constantly run your farm regardless of these changes, but you should know that you can expect higher costs for at least half the year.

Don't Trust Cryptocurrency Holders/Lenders

A great way to ensure your profitability in the future is to hold onto your currency today. This goes for both waiting to sell until there are tell tale signs that you should dump currency, but also that you shouldn't trust banks or any sort of third party service. There have been many banks and similar services popping up for cryptocurrencies, most prominently around Bitcoin. Consistently these services have proven to be absolutely awful at holding onto their customers' money. The service that they offer is depositing your cryptocurrency today and you can borrow against it with real cash. They also claim that by having them hold onto the money you will be able to trade more efficiently, meaning that you can find a quote and initiate an immediate transfer to cash.

There is a fundamental problem in all of these services in that they have proven time and time again to be incredibly unreliable. You are exchanging your cryptocurrency for a username and password that gives you the right to monitor the account. Hackers are quite enthusiastic about breaking into these banks for themselves, and they have consistently done so. In rare cases, the owner of these businesses borrows against the money themselves, and the business goes under because of an inability to pay back loans. There is a lot of temptation of convenience in these services, but don't use them. There is no regulation and there hasn't been a service that has been around long enough to trust on faith alone.

Selling Currency

It's difficult to say exactly how you will realize your profits in the future. The fact that one Bitcoin is worth five hundred dollars does not mean that it can easily be liquefied. The exchanges for cryptocurrencies are ever changing, with competition consistently driving new businesses to pop up. The moment you should start looking for *where* to exchange your currencies is the same moment when you want to change your currencies; you simply can't expect the most favorable exchange to stay the same year over year. My suggestion is that you plan on holding onto any currency that you mine for around five years. This is a good estimate for when you will start to see large returns. You won't know where you will be selling your currency, and you won't know exactly how much it will be worth, but unless a rapid selloff occurs you will want to have some estimation of when you will receive profits. Assume five years as a benchmark and base your financial commitment on the assumption that it will take that long to make your money back.

Chapter 7: Knowing When to Cash Out

It's Almost a Certainty That All Current Cryptocurrencies Will Eventually Fail

Making money through the cryptocurrencies currently on the market is more than possible, it's a certainty. That being said, you must realize that eventually all of the blockchain currencies on today's market will eventually fail. It's not an *absolute* certainty, but the odds are heavy favored against independent blockchain currencies. How this will happen is not going to be a sudden shift; it will be a slow decay in the value and practicality of the currencies. It is going to be in the decline, or just before, that you sell all of your digital currencies. It is therefore predicting the fall of each currency that is going to be the deciding factor in how much profit you can make. This can happen in several different ways, although some scenarios are more likely than others. Before moving onto how currencies will likely fail, let's talk about the unlikely scenario that a currency stays relevant long into the future.

Of all of the currencies on the market, analysts have predicted that if any stay valuable it will come down to two or three major currencies and the rest will fail. Right now the only currency that seems likely to stay relevant far into the future is Bitcoin. Everything else is too new and unproven, either in underlying technologies or because of a lack of faith in the currency by speculators. In a scenario where the currency you mined stays valuable and becomes more and more adopted, you will have an easy time exchanging it for the of a government backed currency. You will know that a currency has become fully adopted once you see a major bank use it in two or more countries. If Bank of America starts allowing deposits of Bitcoin, it's a major step forward, but for real success another major government will have to allow bank branches to allow deposits in another country. There is consensus that this is a sign that a currency is not going to fail. For what it is worth, if this ever happens, I plan on cashing out some portion of my Bitcoins at this time. The value of Bitcoins will surely spike significantly as it becomes known that nearly all vendors will be accepting it, or that it can freely be exchanged for U.S. dollars by simply depositing it in a bank account.

The signs to watch for widespread adoption of a currency are likely not to come from a bank itself, but rather from legislation that allows a bank to hold onto cryptocurrency. You will hear about such legislation months before it ever is approved, and the consequences will be discussed in the media in the lead up to such adoption. This scenario is unlikely, but it will prove to be one of the most profitable. By merely announcing the acceptance of a cryptocurrency, the value will surely skyrocket as more and more speculators get involved.

Government Intervention

The most likely way for blockchain currencies to fail is if a major government issues its own digital currency. This type of event would see most major digital currencies be wiped out over a few short years. A government backed blockchain currency makes all other third party currencies redundant. There will be some that latch onto third party currencies, but if a government issued version has many of the same parameters; that is, functions like digital cash, then it is almost a certainty that all other currencies will become worthless.

Here's what you need to lookout for to make sure that you are not caught in the middle of cryptocurrency devaluation. The moment a small government outside of the

United States adopts a blockchain currency of its own is the first sign that other governments will be considering the same. The reason why the United States likely won't be the first is because its banking system is so robust. For other less developed countries the banking systems are not as strong and fake currency is much more of a problem. It wouldn't be surprising to see India issue a government backed blockchain currency first, since it would address the country's goals of reducing counterfeit money and improving where electronic payment is accepted.

When you start to see that a foreign country has adopted blockchain technologies, it's time to start preparing how you are going to dump your currency. The institutions for exchange will likely be different than they are today, but you will want to dump at least half of your holdings. How much you decide to keep is going to be based on how confident you are that the currency will rise again before it gets completely taken over by a government currency.

Security Failure at a System Level

You know a bit about blockchain technology, and why it has proven to be useful for creating a secure form of currency that works because each individual in the system has full access to all of the information about changes in the currency. If this security measure were to ever fail, the underlying currency would be knocked out entirely. This is a worst case scenario for investors of blockchain currencies. If a miner found a way to create an infinite number of Bitcoins for themselves, the moment the news got out the entire currency would be worthless. I don't think that this is a likely scenario, but it is the reason why I would invest in more than one currency. To be clear, blockchain currencies have seen widespread adoption because of how secure they are – this is

51

an unlikely scenario but one you can easily protect yourself against, and so you should.

A Major Institution Develops and Is Subsequently destroyed

Of the services that will hold onto Bitcoins, most have either fallen or have come with a less than perfect reputation. So far the number of institutions that have popped up is quite large, and so the failure of any one institution will not mean the currency is destroyed entirely. It is possible that a major institution will come to prominence in the future, and for several examples, you must only look to Bitcoin. There have been several large 'banks' that have developed around Bitcoin. They were convenient for deposits, and the ability to convert Bitcoin to traditional currencies immediately was seen as a huge benefit. When these companies fail the faith behind the currency it held is severely damaged. So far no one institution has garnered enough of the market for it to wipe out a currency, but that scenario is far from unlikely.

What you will want to watch out for is if a single group comes to be the predominate holder of a blockchain currency. If this ever happens, I would sell some portion of my holdings. It will be tempting to hold onto the currency as you will likely see its value rise with the success of such a company, but in the off chance that the company falters, you will want to have sold off some of your holdings already. At the very least, you want to have your hand on the pulse of that company, ensuring that if any problems arise, you will be among the first to cash out.

Conclusion

Thank you again for purchasing *Blockchain: How to Use the Hidden Economy to Your Advantage.*

I hope this book has helped you learn how to earn profit with cryptocurrencies and blockchain technology. You now have the essential knowledge that you need to get started. You know why blockchain currencies rise in value, the trouble spots to look out for, and you even know how to get started mining a variety of different currencies yourself.

Your next step is to start building the computers that you will use for mining, and then decide what currencies you want to mine. Make sure that you mine at least two currencies, referring to chapter three for a reminder about the preferred currencies you will want to obtain. Be sure to build your mining computers yourself. The process of building your own computer is quite easy, and the savings you achieve in building your own mining computers are immense. Use the right cooling paste and keep the power supply and heat from your mining computers in mind. Remember that you will be fighting against electricity, and this is the primary factor that will cut into your profits. Try and minimize the total cost of energy by sourcing the parts that I described in chapter five. Always go for the best power to wattage ratio, and make sure that unnecessary devices for a computer are never kept plugged in, such as monitors.

Your final step to profitability will be selling the blockchain currencies that you mine. You know what signs to lookout for, and as long as you are paying attention to the market, you will be able to cash out at the right time. It is a long road to maximum profitability with blockchain currencies, but remember that you are free to cash out at any time. I have done this several times in the past to put money in my pocket, oftentimes for reinvesting into more mining machines. Do what is best for you and your specific financial situation, but always try and get as much as you can for the cryptocurrencies that you mine.

Lastly if you enjoyed this book, it would be much appreciated if you could leave a review on Amazon. The best way for this book to make its way into the hands of more readers is through truthful reviews about this work. Please write what you liked about this book and what could be improved upon. Any and all feedback is helpful as I continue to serve the needs of my readership.

Thank you and good luck!

Made in the USA
Coppell, TX
28 October 2020